# CHAIR YOGA FOR WEIGHT LOSS

Gentle Workouts for Effective Fat Burning to
Transform Your Body with Easy Seated Exercises

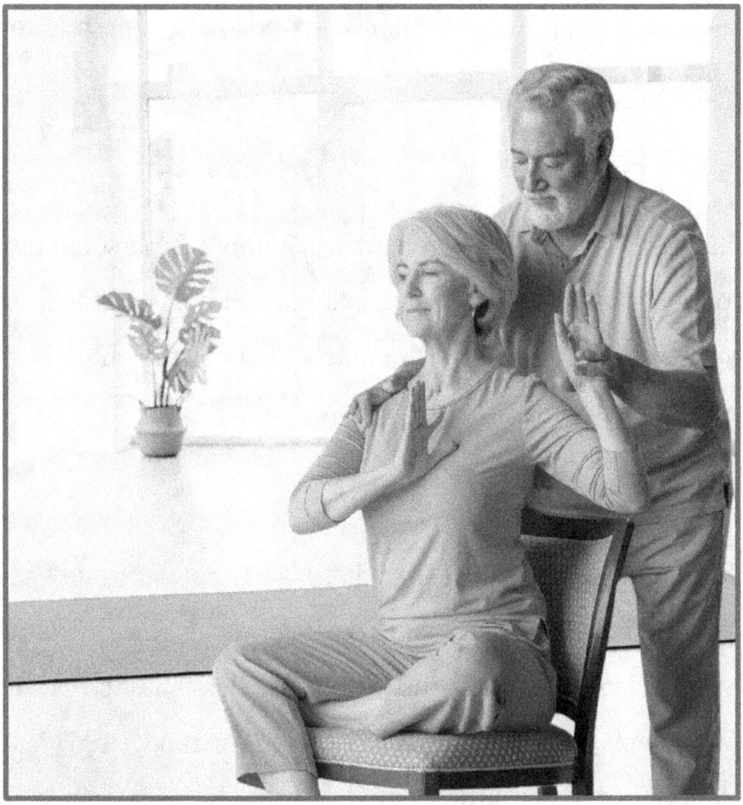

## HARRY LAVELLE

# TABLE OF CONTENT

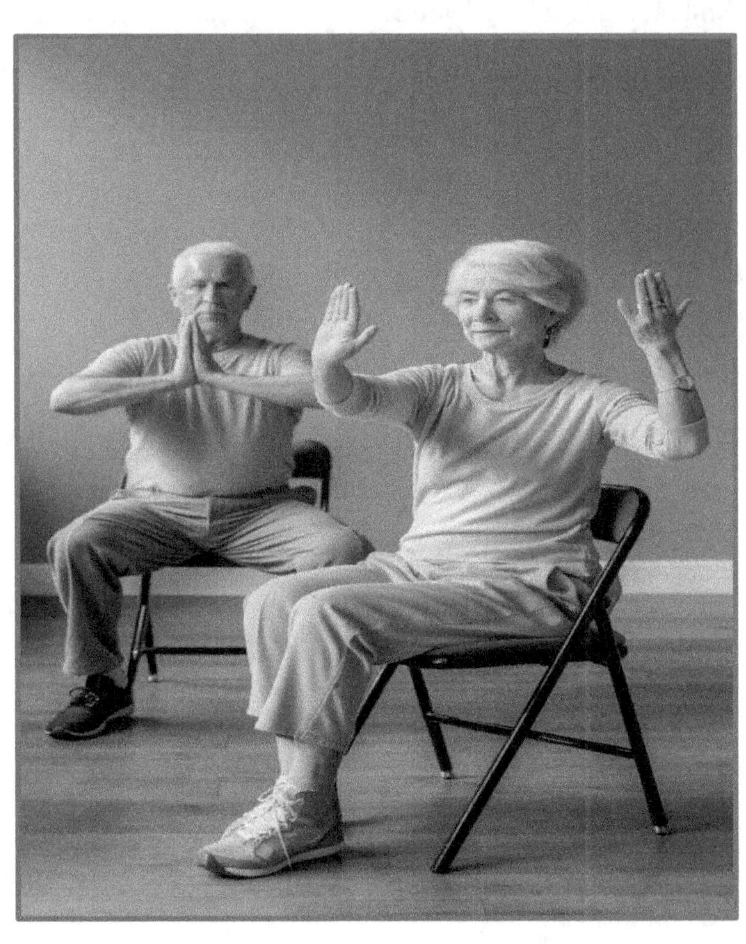

# INTRODUCTION

Have you ever looked at the person across from you at the dinner table and thought, "We've got to do something about this"? Maybe those late-night snacks have turned into a permanent fixture, or the simple act of bending over to tie your shoes now feels like a workout. It was exactly this way for Mike and Sarah. They were two people trapped in a cycle of lethargy, their love for each other overshadowed by their growing waistlines and the creeping despair that came with each failed diet.

**Mike, a once-active software developer, now spent his days hunched over a keyboard**, his belly pressing against his desk. Sarah, a vibrant kindergarten teacher, found herself exhausted before the school day even began, her energy zapped by the extra weight she carried. They both knew they needed a change, but the thought of another gym membership or restrictive diet plan filled them with dread.

Then, a chance encounter with a forgotten book tucked away in their attic changed everything. "Chair Yoga for Weight Loss" – a title that initially made them chuckle, but one that held the promise of a solution that was both gentle and effective. At first, they were skeptical. How could a few simple stretches in a chair possibly make a difference? But with nothing to lose, they decided to give it a try.

What followed was a transformation that neither of them could have predicted. The chair yoga routines, initially a source of amusement, became a daily ritual they both looked forward to. The gentle movements not only helped them shed pounds, but also ignited a spark of joy they hadn't felt in years. Mike found himself standing taller, his confidence returning with each downward dog. Sarah's energy soared, her laughter echoing through the classroom once again.

But this book isn't just about Mike and Sarah. It's about you, and the incredible potential that lies dormant within your body. It's about discovering a path to weight loss that doesn't involve deprivation or exhaustion, but rather, a reawakening of your inner strength and vitality.

**If you're tired of fad diets and grueling workouts, if you're ready to embrace a path that's both sustainable and enjoyable,** then this book is for you. I promise you, the results you'll achieve will be far more profound than a number on a scale. You'll rediscover the joy of movement, the confidence that comes with a healthy body, and the unwavering belief in your own ability to create lasting change.

Don't wait another day to embark on this life-changing journey. Turn the page, and let the magic of chair yoga transform your life, just as it did for Mike and Sarah. Your healthier, happier self awaits.

**Are you ready to begin?**

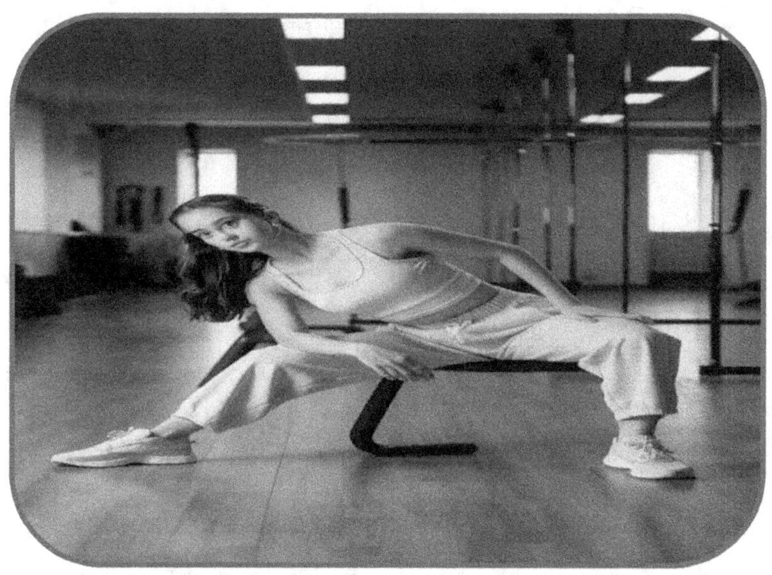

## The Role of Chair Yoga

Chair yoga offers an accessible pathway to wellness, especially for those seeking a gentle yet effective way to enhance their physical and mental health. By incorporating simple, seated poses and mindful breathing, chair yoga adapts traditional yoga practices to accommodate various abilities and fitness levels.

Imagine a practice that transforms your living room or office into a sanctuary of calm. Chair yoga makes this possible, requiring only a chair and a bit of space. It allows individuals with mobility issues, seniors, or those new to exercise to experience the benefits of yoga without the intimidation of floor-based poses.

The beauty of chair yoga lies in its versatility. It strengthens muscles, improves flexibility, and enhances balance, all while reducing stress and anxiety. Regular practice can lead to better posture, increased circulation, and a greater sense of well-being.

For those embarking on a weight loss journey, chair yoga complements other activities by promoting mindfulness and body awareness, helping you make healthier choices. It's a gentle reminder that movement and wellness are achievable at any stage of life.

Incorporate chair yoga into your routine and discover a rejuvenating practice that nurtures both body and mind, empowering you to embrace a healthier, more balanced lifestyle.

# CHAPTER 1

# FOUNDATIONS OF CHAIR YOGA

## What is Chair Yoga?

Chair yoga is a gentle form of yoga practiced while seated or using a chair for support, making it accessible to people of all ages and fitness levels. This adaptation allows individuals with mobility challenges, seniors, or those new to yoga to experience its numerous benefits without the need for floor-based poses.

**Incorporating traditional yoga postures, breathing techniques, and meditation,** chair yoga enhances flexibility, strength, and balance. It's a versatile practice that can be done anywhere—at home, in the office, or even while traveling—requiring only a chair and a little space.

The beauty of chair yoga lies in its ability to bring the profound benefits of yoga to everyone. It reduces stress, improves mental clarity, and promotes a sense of calm and well-being. For those on a weight loss journey, chair yoga also encourages mindful movement and body awareness, supporting healthier lifestyle choices.

By integrating chair yoga into your routine, you embrace a holistic approach to health that nurtures both body and mind, empowering you to live a more balanced and fulfilling life. Discover the transformative power of chair yoga and unlock a path to improved wellness and vitality.

## Key Benefits for Weight Loss

Chair yoga offers a unique and accessible approach to weight loss, making it ideal for individuals of all fitness levels. By engaging in gentle movements and mindful breathing, it helps increase metabolism and burn calories effectively. Each session enhances flexibility, strength, and balance, contributing to a more active lifestyle.

**This practice promotes body awareness, encouraging healthier eating habits and fostering a positive relationship with food.** By reducing stress and anxiety, chair yoga helps curb emotional eating, which can be a significant barrier to weight loss.

Regular participation in chair yoga boosts energy levels, making it easier to stay motivated and committed to your weight loss journey. Additionally, the improved circulation and muscle tone aid in better digestion and fat burning.

Incorporating chair yoga into your routine provides a holistic approach to weight management, supporting both physical and mental well-being. Embrace this gentle yet powerful practice to achieve your weight loss goals and enhance your overall quality of life.

## Busting Myths

Chair yoga is often misunderstood, yet it offers remarkable benefits for weight loss and overall health. Contrary to popular belief, chair yoga is not just for seniors or those with limited mobility; it's a versatile practice that anyone can incorporate into their fitness routine.

One common myth is that chair yoga is too easy to be effective. However, this gentle form of exercise builds strength, flexibility, and balance, engaging core muscles and boosting metabolism. Each session can burn calories and improve circulation, making it an effective tool for weight management.

Another misconception is that chair yoga lacks intensity. In reality, the practice encourages mindfulness and breath control, which enhance mental focus and stress reduction. By calming the mind and reducing cortisol levels, chair yoga helps prevent stress-related weight gain.

Embrace chair yoga as a legitimate and powerful addition to your fitness regimen. It offers a holistic approach, addressing both physical and emotional well-being. Discover the truth about chair yoga and unlock its potential to transform your weight loss journey.

# CHAPTER 2

# SCIENTIFIC INSIGHTS

## How Chair Yoga Aids Weight Loss

Chair yoga is a powerful tool for those seeking to lose weight, offering a gentle yet effective approach to fitness. Unlike traditional exercises, chair yoga provides a unique blend of accessibility and efficacy, making it suitable for all fitness levels.

### Boosting Metabolism

One of the key benefits of chair yoga is its ability to boost metabolism. Through a series of dynamic poses and stretches, chair yoga stimulates muscle activity, which in turn increases the metabolic rate. This process helps the body burn calories more efficiently, even during rest. By incorporating movements that engage the core, arms, and legs, chair yoga promotes muscle toning and strength, essential components for effective weight loss.

## Enhancing Flexibility and Balance

Improved flexibility and balance are crucial for maintaining an active lifestyle. Chair yoga stretches and lengthens muscles, reducing stiffness and increasing range of motion. This enhancement allows for more active participation in various physical activities, contributing to increased calorie expenditure. Additionally, improved balance reduces the risk of injuries, encouraging consistent exercise routines.

## Stress Reduction

Stress is a significant barrier to weight loss, often leading to emotional eating and weight gain. Chair yoga incorporates mindfulness and deep breathing techniques, which are powerful tools for stress reduction. By calming the mind and lowering cortisol levels, it helps prevent stress-related weight gain. Practicing mindfulness also encourages better eating habits, fostering a more conscious approach to nutrition.

## Improving Circulation

Chair yoga enhances blood flow, ensuring that nutrients are effectively distributed throughout the body. Improved circulation supports overall health, helping organs function optimally and promoting detoxification. This increased efficiency aids in the removal of waste products, which can contribute to weight gain if left unchecked.

**Encouraging Consistency**

One of the most significant advantages of chair yoga is its accessibility. It can be practiced anywhere, requiring minimal equipment and space. This ease of practice encourages consistency, which is crucial for weight loss. Regular sessions can be seamlessly integrated into daily routines, ensuring that physical activity becomes a sustainable habit.

**Building Mind-Body Connection**

Chair yoga emphasizes the mind-body connection, fostering a deeper awareness of bodily sensations and movements. This connection encourages individuals to listen to their bodies and make healthier choices. By cultivating this awareness, chair yoga empowers practitioners to respond to their body's needs, such as recognizing hunger and satiety cues, which are vital for weight management.

**Customizable Workouts**

Chair yoga offers a versatile approach that can be tailored to individual needs and fitness levels. Whether you're a beginner or an experienced yogi, chair yoga can be adapted to challenge and inspire you. This customization ensures that your practice remains engaging and effective, preventing plateaus in your weight loss journey.

Incorporating chair yoga into your lifestyle is a transformative step toward achieving weight loss goals. Its holistic approach addresses not only the physical aspects of fitness but also the mental and emotional barriers that often hinder progress. Embrace chair yoga as a supportive companion on your journey to a healthier, more balanced life.

## Research and Evidence

Chair yoga is backed by a growing body of research highlighting its benefits for weight loss and overall health. Studies have shown that chair yoga can significantly improve flexibility, strength, and balance, which are essential for maintaining an active lifestyle. This gentle form of exercise has been proven to increase metabolic rates, helping the body burn calories more efficiently.

In addition, research indicates that chair yoga reduces stress and anxiety, both of which are closely linked to weight gain. By incorporating mindfulness and deep breathing techniques, chair yoga helps lower cortisol levels, promoting a sense of calm and reducing emotional eating.

Clinical trials have also demonstrated that regular practice of chair yoga enhances cardiovascular health by improving circulation and lowering blood pressure. These benefits contribute to a healthier metabolism and aid in weight management.

The accessibility and adaptability of chair yoga make it an ideal choice for seniors and those with mobility challenges. It provides a safe and effective way to engage in physical activity, ensuring that everyone can experience the transformative effects of yoga. By incorporating evidence-based practices, chair yoga offers a holistic approach to achieving weight loss and wellness goals.

## Case Studies and Testimonials

### Transformative Stories of Chair Yoga Success

In recent years, chair yoga has emerged as a powerful tool for those seeking a gentle yet effective approach to weight loss and wellness. The real-life experiences of individuals who have embraced chair yoga offer compelling evidence of its transformative potential.

### Mary's Journey to Wellness

Mary, a 68-year-old retiree, struggled with joint pain and limited mobility, which made traditional exercise difficult. After discovering chair yoga, she began attending classes twice a week. Within months, Mary noticed significant improvements in her flexibility and balance. She felt more energetic and experienced a gradual but steady weight loss. Her story is a testament to how chair yoga can empower seniors to reclaim their health and vitality.

Mary shares, "Chair yoga gave me my life back. I never thought I could enjoy exercise again, but now I look forward to each session."

**Tom's Path to a Healthier Lifestyle**

Tom, a 55-year-old office worker, found himself in a cycle of stress and weight gain due to his sedentary job. Intrigued by the low-impact nature of chair yoga, he decided to try it during his lunch breaks. Over time, Tom not only lost weight but also noticed a significant reduction in his stress levels. The practice helped him reconnect with his body and develop healthier habits.

"Chair yoga was the missing piece in my wellness puzzle," Tom explains. "It's helped me manage my weight and stress, making a huge difference in my overall quality of life."

**Linda's Testimonial of Change**

Linda, a 72-year-old grandmother, wanted to improve her health to keep up with her grandchildren. She was hesitant to start any exercise routine due to chronic back pain. A friend recommended chair yoga as a gentle alternative. After participating in a local class, Linda quickly experienced relief from her pain and gained strength she thought was lost forever.

"Chair yoga has been a revelation," Linda says. "I'm now more active with my family, and the weight loss has been an amazing bonus."

**The Impact of Community Support**

These testimonials highlight the power of community in chair yoga classes. Participants often find a sense of camaraderie and support, which enhances their commitment to regular practice. This supportive environment fosters accountability and encourages personal growth.

**The Science Behind the Success**

These success stories are backed by scientific research showing that chair yoga enhances physical and mental well-being. Its focus on breath control and mindfulness helps reduce stress, a major factor in weight management. Additionally, the gentle movements improve circulation and metabolism, supporting a healthy weight loss journey.

**A Promising Future**

The compelling narratives of Mary, Tom, and Linda illustrate the diverse benefits of chair yoga. As more people share their experiences, the popularity of this accessible form of exercise continues to grow. Whether for weight loss, improved mobility, or enhanced mental clarity, chair yoga offers a pathway to a healthier, more fulfilling life.

By incorporating chair yoga into their routines, individuals are discovering renewed confidence and a better quality of life. These stories remind us that it's never too late to embark on a journey toward wellness and self-discovery.

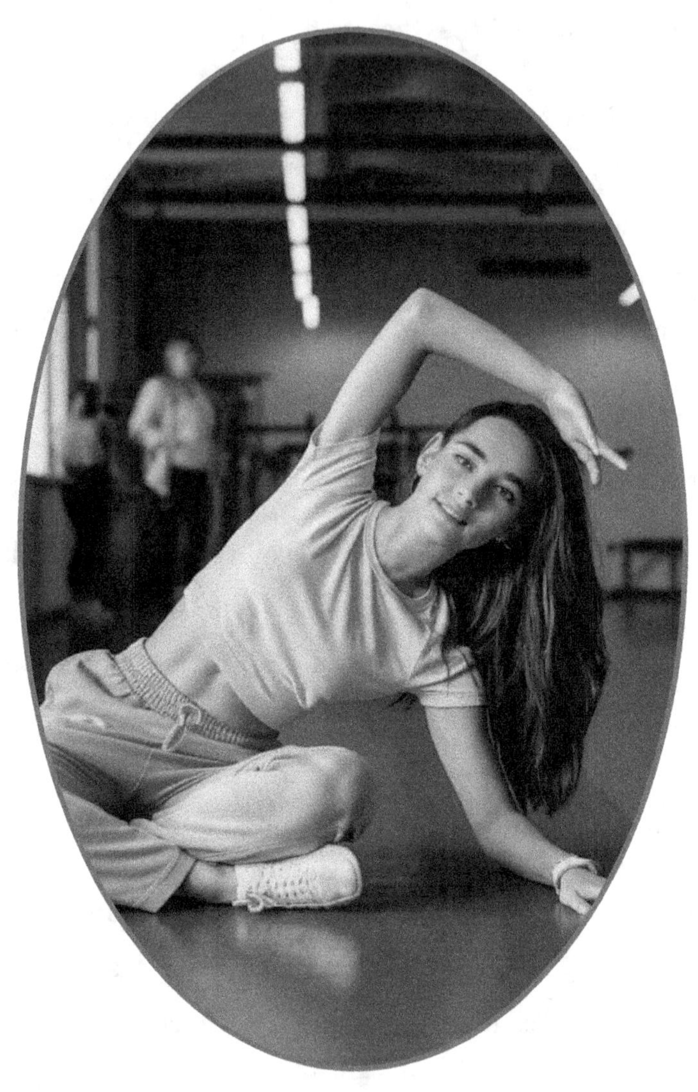

# CHAPTER 3

# ESSENTIAL CHAIR YOGA POSES

## Beginner-Friendly Poses

Chair yoga offers a welcoming entry point for anyone seeking the benefits of yoga without the strain of traditional practices. It's particularly appealing to beginners, providing a gentle yet effective way to enhance flexibility, strength, and overall well-being.

Making it ideal for individuals with limited mobility or those recovering from injuries. The support of a chair allows practitioners to perform poses safely and comfortably, reducing the risk of strain or injury.

- **Increased Flexibility**: Regular practice improves joint mobility and muscle flexibility.

- **Enhanced Strength**: Builds muscle strength gradually, supporting better posture and balance.

- **Stress Reduction**: Encourages mindfulness and relaxation, reducing stress and anxiety.

**Essential Poses for Beginners**

**1. Seated Mountain Pose (Tadasana)**

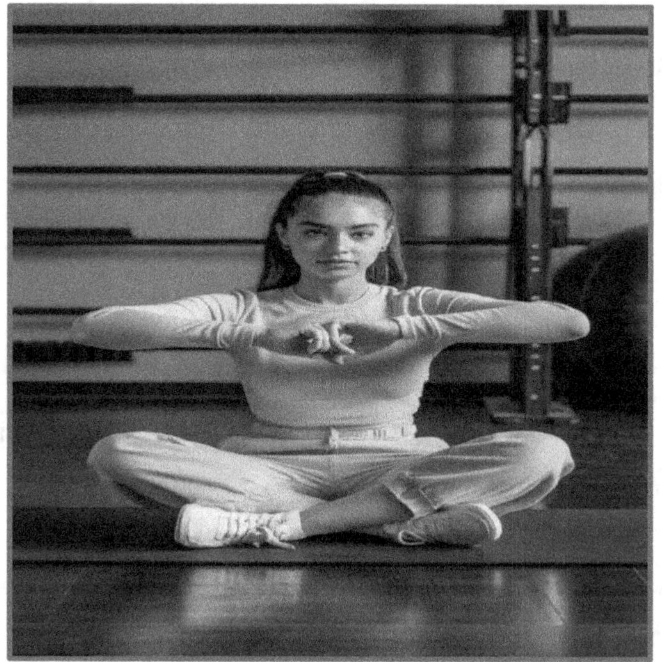

- **How to Do It**: Sit up straight with feet flat on the floor. Keep your spine aligned, shoulders relaxed, and arms at your sides or on your lap.

- **Benefits**: Encourages proper posture and enhances awareness of alignment.

## 2. Seated Forward Bend (Paschimottanasana)

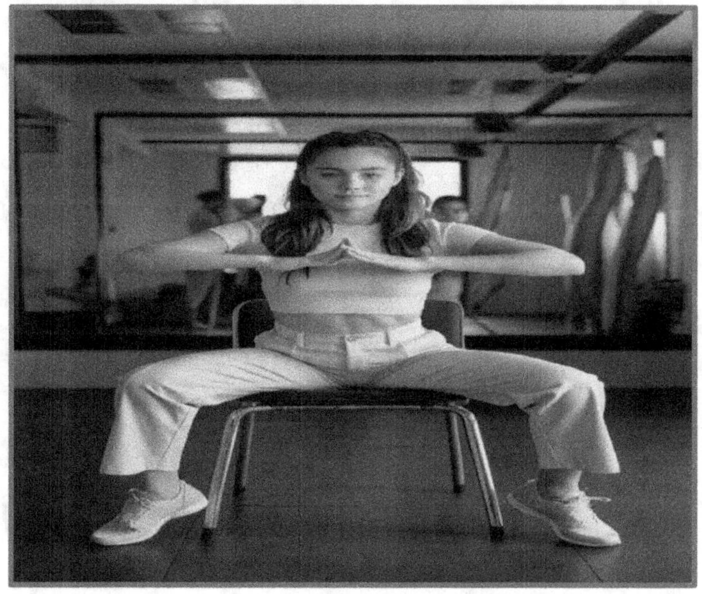

- **How to Do It**: From a seated position, slowly bend forward, reaching towards your toes. Keep your spine long and only go as far as comfortable.

- **Benefits**: Stretches the back and hamstrings, promoting relaxation and flexibility.

### 3.  Chair Cat-Cow Stretch

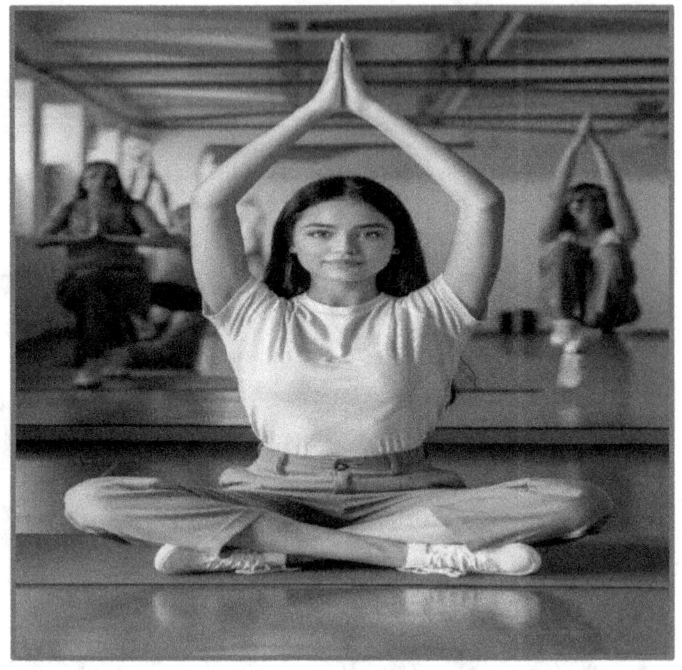

- **How to Do It**: Sit with hands on knees. Inhale, arch your back (cow), and look up. Exhale, round your spine (cat), and tuck your chin.

- **Benefits**: Improves spinal flexibility and relieves tension in the back.

## 4. Seated Side Bend

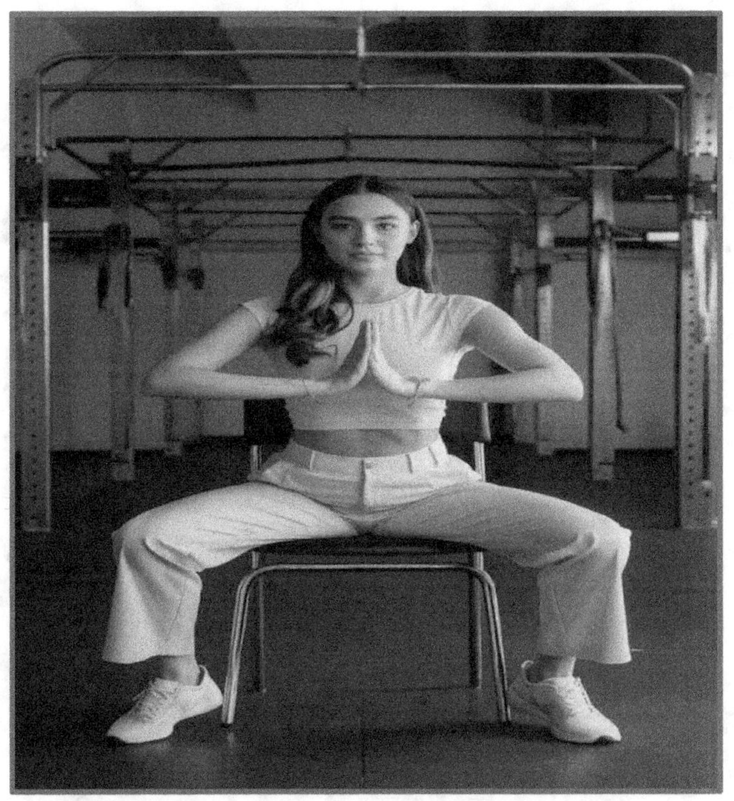

- **How to Do It**: Sit tall, raise one arm overhead, and gently lean to the opposite side. Hold and switch sides.

- **Benefits**: Stretches the sides of the body, enhancing flexibility and relieving tension.

## 5.  Chair Pigeon Pose

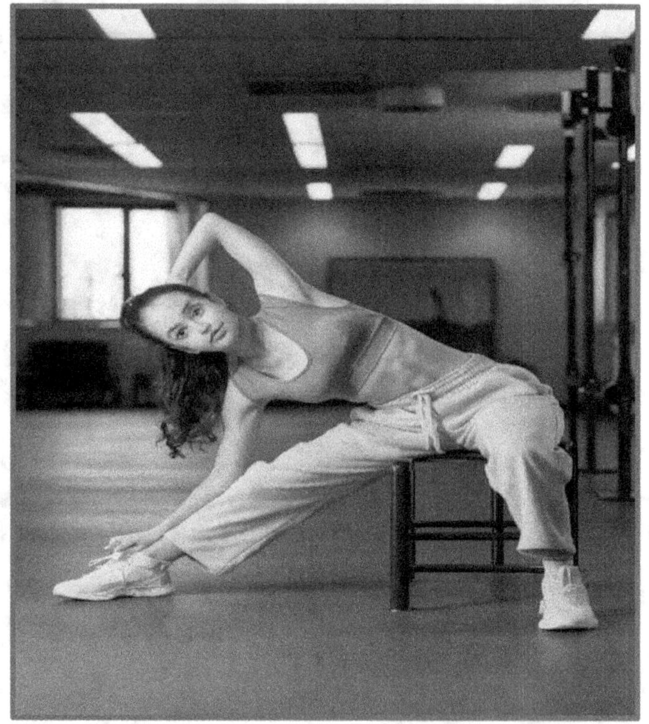

- **How to Do It**: Cross one ankle over the opposite knee, sitting up tall. Gently press the crossed knee downwards for a deeper stretch.

- **Benefits**: Opens hips and stretches glutes, aiding in hip mobility.

**Tips for a Successful Practice**

- **Focus on Breath**: Breathing deeply and steadily enhances the benefits of each pose.

- **Listen to Your Body**: Move at your own pace and modify poses to suit your comfort level.

- **Consistency is Key**: Regular practice leads to gradual improvements in strength and flexibility.

**Encouragement for Beginners**

Starting with chair yoga provides a foundation for building confidence in your yoga practice. It's a reminder that yoga is for everyone, regardless of age or physical ability. As you become familiar with these beginner-friendly poses, you'll find yourself progressing naturally, opening the door to more advanced movements.

Chair yoga's simplicity and accessibility make it a perfect choice for those new to yoga or seeking a gentle approach to physical activity. By incorporating these beginner-friendly poses into your routine, you're taking a significant step toward improved health and well-being.

Embark on this journey with an open heart, knowing that each pose is a building block toward greater strength, flexibility, and inner peace. Embrace the process, and enjoy the many benefits that chair yoga has to offer.

## Detailed Instructions and Modifications

Chair yoga offers an accessible way to experience the benefits of yoga, especially for those with limited mobility. The key is understanding how to modify poses to suit individual needs, ensuring both safety and effectiveness.

### Starting with the Basics

Before diving into specific poses, it's essential to establish a solid foundation:

- **Posture Awareness**: Sit with feet flat on the floor, back straight, and shoulders relaxed. This posture forms the basis for most chair yoga poses.

- **Breath Control**: Focus on deep, steady breaths. Inhale through the nose and exhale through the mouth, synchronizing with movements.

**Essential Poses and Modifications**

**1. Seated Mountain Pose (Tad asana)**

- **Instructions**: Sit tall, feet hip-width apart. Extend arms overhead or rest them on your lap.

- **Modification**: If raising arms is challenging, keep hands on thighs to focus on posture.

**2. Chair Forward Bend (Uttanasana)**

- **Instructions**: From a seated position, hinge at the hips and reach toward your feet, keeping the spine long.

- **Modification**: Use a strap around the feet for support, or rest hands on knees if reaching forward is difficult.

## 3. Seated Twist (Ardha Matsyendrasana)

- **Instructions**: Sit upright, place one hand on the opposite knee, and twist gently to the side.

- **Modification**: Keep the twist mild, moving only as far as comfortable without straining the neck.

## 4. Leg Lifts

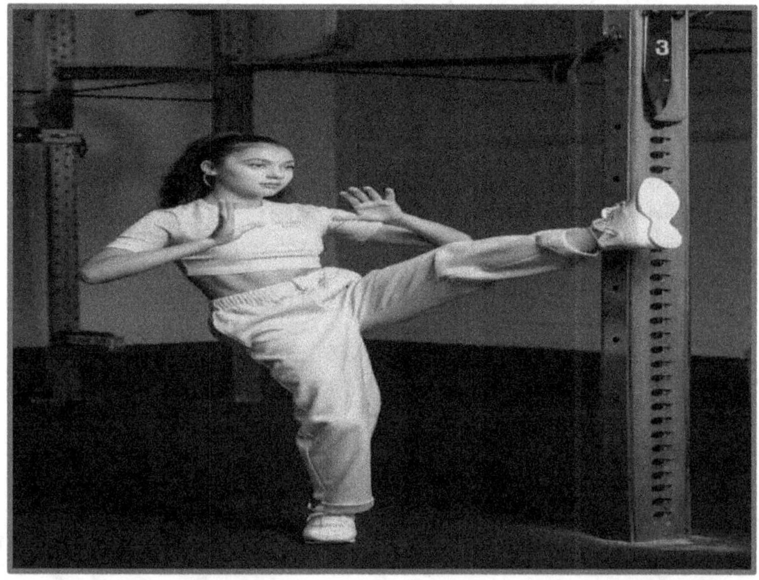

- **Instructions**: Sit with back straight, lift one leg parallel to the floor, hold, and lower.

- **Modification**: If lifting the leg is difficult, keep the heel on the ground and slide it forward and back.

## 5. Chair Warrior Pose (Virabhadrasana)

- **Instructions**: Sit sideways on the chair, extend one leg back, and raise arms overhead.

- **Modification**: Keep the back foot on the ground with a slight bend in the knee for added stability.

## Tips for Successful Modifications

- **Listen to Your Body**: Pay attention to any discomfort or pain, and adjust poses accordingly.

- **Use Props**: Incorporate straps, blocks, or cushions to enhance stability and comfort.

- **Progress Gradually**: Start with simpler modifications and gradually attempt more challenging variations as confidence grows.

## Benefits of Modifying Poses

- **Increased Accessibility**: Modifications make yoga inclusive, allowing everyone to participate regardless of physical limitations.

- **Enhanced Safety**: Adapting poses reduces the risk of injury and encourages a sustainable practice.

- **Personalized Practice**: Tailor yoga to meet individual goals and abilities, creating a more fulfilling experience.

## Encouragement for Practitioners

Embrace the journey of chair yoga with an open mind. Every modification is an opportunity to learn more about your body and its capabilities. Celebrate each small victory, knowing that consistent practice leads to improved strength, flexibility, and peace of mind.

Chair yoga, with its adaptable nature, empowers individuals to enjoy the transformative benefits of yoga. By mastering detailed instructions and modifications, you'll gain confidence in your practice and unlock the potential for lifelong wellness. Remember, yoga is not about perfection—it's about progress and self-discovery.

Start today, and allow chair yoga to guide you toward a healthier, more vibrant life.

## Safety Tips and Precautions

Chair yoga is a wonderful way to enjoy the benefits of yoga, especially for seniors or those with limited mobility. To ensure a safe and enjoyable practice, it's important to follow certain safety tips and precautions.

**Understanding Your Body**

1. **Know Your Limits**: Listen to your body. It's crucial to understand your physical boundaries and avoid pushing beyond them.

2. **Respect Pain Signals**: Yoga should never cause pain. If you feel discomfort, gently ease out of the pose and rest.

**Creating a Safe Environment**

1. **Stable Chair**: Use a sturdy chair without wheels. Ensure it's placed on a non-slip surface to prevent any movement during practice.

2. **Adequate Space**: Clear the area around your chair to allow for free movement of arms and legs without obstruction.

**Warm-Up and Cool Down**

1. **Begin with Warm-Ups**: Start with gentle movements to warm up your muscles. This helps prevent strain or injury.

2. **End with Relaxation**: Cool down with deep breathing or meditation to help your body relax and integrate the practice.

## Proper Attire

1. **Comfortable Clothing**: Wear loose, stretchy clothing that allows full range of motion without restriction.

2. **Barefoot or Non-Slip Shoes**: Practice barefoot for better grip, or use non-slip shoes if you need extra stability.

## Hydration and Nutrition

1. **Stay Hydrated**: Drink water before and after your session to keep your body hydrated.

2. **Light Meals**: Avoid heavy meals before practicing yoga. Opt for a light snack if needed.

## Using Props

1. **Supportive Props**: Use yoga blocks, straps, or cushions to assist in achieving poses comfortably.

2. **Wall Support**: Perform exercises near a wall for added support and balance if necessary.

## Techniques for Safe Practice

1. **Controlled Movements**: Move slowly and deliberately into each pose, focusing on control rather than speed.

2. **Mindful Breathing**: Coordinate your breath with movements. Inhale during expansion and exhale during contraction.

## Modifying Poses

1. **Adapt to Your Needs**: Modify poses based on your abilities. It's perfectly fine to adjust movements to fit your comfort level.

2. **Consult a Professional**: If you're unsure about a pose, consult with a yoga instructor to ensure proper alignment and technique.

## Medical Considerations

1. **Consult Your Doctor**: If you have any medical
   conditions or concerns, consult with a healthcare
   professional before beginning a yoga practice.

2. **Monitor Health Conditions**: Keep track of how
   your body responds, especially if you have
   conditions like arthritis or hypertension.

## Mindful Practice

1. **Focus on the Present**: Practice mindfulness by
   focusing on your breath and movements. This
   enhances both safety and the mental benefits of
   yoga.

2. **Regular Check-Ins**: Periodically assess how your
   body feels during the session, adjusting as needed.

## Encouragement and Support

1. **Progress at Your Own Pace**: Yoga is a personal
   journey. Celebrate small achievements and be
   patient with your progress.

2. **Join a Community**: Consider joining a chair yoga class or group to receive guidance and encouragement.

# CHAPTER 4

# DESIGNING YOUR PRACTICE

## Creating Effective chair yoga Routines

Designing effective chair yoga routines is essential for achieving fitness goals, especially for seniors seeking improved health and wellness. Here's how to create routines that are engaging, safe, and beneficial.

**Understanding Your Goals**

1. **Define Your Objectives**: Determine what you want to achieve—whether it's increasing flexibility, enhancing strength, or relieving stress.

2. **Set Realistic Expectations**: Understand your current fitness level and set achievable goals to keep motivation high.

**Structuring Your Routine**

1. **Warm-Up**: Begin with gentle movements to prepare the body. Simple neck rolls, shoulder shrugs, and ankle circles help loosen muscles and joints.

2. **Core Sequence**: Focus on poses that address your specific goals. Include a mix of stretching, strengthening, and balancing exercises.

3. **Cool Down**: End with calming exercises like seated meditation or deep breathing to help your body relax and recover.

**Selecting Poses**

1. **Variety is Key**: Incorporate a range of poses to target different muscle groups. Use stretches for flexibility and strength-building exercises to enhance muscle tone.

2. **Adaptability**: Choose poses that can be easily modified to suit various ability levels, ensuring accessibility for all participants.

## Incorporating Breathing Techniques

1. **Mindful Breathing**: Integrate breathing exercises to enhance relaxation and focus. Teach deep, diaphragmatic breathing to support each movement.

2. **Breath Coordination**: Align breath with movement to increase the effectiveness of the practice. Inhale to expand, exhale to release.

## Maintaining Engagement

1. **Keep It Dynamic**: Rotate different routines to prevent monotony and keep the practice exciting and engaging.

2. **Use Music and Visualization**: Enhance the experience with calming music or guided visualizations to create a soothing atmosphere.

## Personalizing Your Practice

1. **Tailor to Needs**: Modify routines based on personal preferences or physical conditions. Customize sessions to accommodate varying energy levels and moods.

2. **Feedback Loop**: Encourage self-assessment and adjustments. Listen to your body and refine routines based on feedback.

## Monitoring Progress

1. **Track Achievements**: Keep a journal to document improvements and challenges. Celebrate milestones to maintain motivation.

2. **Adjust as Needed**: Evaluate your progress regularly and modify routines to meet evolving goals and capabilities.

## Safety Considerations

1. **Prioritize Safety**: Ensure each pose is performed with proper alignment to avoid injury. Use props like blocks and straps for support.

2. **Consult Professionals**: If unsure about any exercises, seek guidance from a certified yoga instructor to ensure correct technique.

**Encouraging Consistency**

1. **Routine Schedule**: Set a regular practice schedule to establish consistency. Even short daily sessions can lead to significant benefits over time.

2. **Accountability Partners**: Practice with a friend or join a group to stay motivated and committed.

## Tailoring to Personal Needs

Personalizing your chair yoga practice ensures that it aligns with your unique physical and emotional requirements. By customizing exercises, you can maximize benefits and enjoy a fulfilling experience.

**Understanding Individual Differences**

1. **Physical Condition**: Assess your current health status, including any limitations or areas of concern, such as joint pain or muscle stiffness.

2. **Fitness Goals**: Define what you want to achieve— be it weight loss, improved flexibility, or stress relief. Having clear objectives guides your practice.

## Adapting Poses for Comfort

1. **Modify as Needed**: Adjust poses to suit your range of motion. For example, use a cushion to support your back or a strap to extend your reach.

2. **Focus on Alignment**: Proper alignment prevents injuries and enhances effectiveness. Adjust seating positions to maintain correct posture.

## Incorporating Props

1. **Use Props Wisely**: Utilize blocks, straps, and cushions to aid in achieving poses comfortably. They provide stability and ease, especially for beginners.

2. **Experiment with Support**: Discover which props enhance your practice. For instance, a block under the feet can help with balance in certain poses.

## Listening to Your Body

1. **Mindful Awareness**: Pay attention to how your body feels during each session. Adjust intensity based on your energy levels and comfort.

2. **Respect Limits**: Avoid pushing past your boundaries. Yoga should be a gentle, nurturing practice that respects your body's signals.

**Personalizing Breathing Techniques**

1. **Find Your Rhythm**: Experiment with different breathing exercises to discover what calms and centers you best.

2. **Synchronize Breath with Movement**: Use your breath to guide and deepen your practice, enhancing focus and relaxation.

**Addressing Emotional Needs**

1. **Cultivate Mindfulness**: Incorporate meditation or mindfulness practices to support emotional well-being. This fosters a holistic approach to health.

2. **Create a Calming Environment**: Set up your practice space with soothing elements like soft lighting and calming scents.

## Adjusting for Progress

1. **Track Progress**: Maintain a journal to note improvements and areas needing attention. Reflect on achievements to motivate continued growth.

2. **Evolve Your Practice**: As you progress, introduce new poses or increase intensity to keep challenging yourself and avoid plateaus.

## Building a Routine

1. **Consistency is Key**: Establish a regular schedule that fits your lifestyle. Consistency leads to better results and a stronger habit.

2. **Flexible Timing**: Adapt your practice duration based on daily availability, ensuring it remains a stress-free part of your routine.

## Encouraging Self-Reflection

1. **Regular Check-ins**: Periodically assess your goals and practice to ensure they align with your changing needs and abilities.

2. **Celebrate Milestones**: Acknowledge your achievements, no matter how small, to maintain enthusiasm and commitment.

**Seeking Professional Guidance**

1. **Consult Instructors**: If possible, work with a yoga instructor to receive personalized advice and adjustments.

2. **Access Resources**: Utilize books, videos, and online classes to gain new insights and enhance your practice.

# Setting Realistic Goals for Chair Yoga

Setting achievable goals is crucial for a successful chair yoga journey, especially when aiming for weight loss and improved well-being. Here's how to set and reach your objectives effectively.

**Understanding the Importance of Goals**

1. **Clarity and Focus**: Clear goals provide direction and motivation. They help you prioritize and stay committed to your practice.

2. **Measurable Progress**: Defined objectives allow you to track improvements, keeping you engaged and motivated over time.

**Steps to Setting Realistic Goals**

1. **Assess Your Starting Point**: Understand your current fitness level, flexibility, and any physical limitations. This will help set goals that are challenging yet attainable.

2. **Define Specific Objectives**: Instead of vague goals like "get fit," aim for specific targets such as "increase flexibility in the hips" or "practice chair yoga three times a week."

3. **Set Short and Long-term Goals**: Balance immediate objectives with future aspirations. Short-term goals provide quick wins, while long-term ones keep you focused on sustained progress.

## Making Goals Achievable

1. **Be Honest with Yourself**: Consider your schedule, lifestyle, and commitments when setting goals. Avoid over-ambitious targets that may lead to frustration.

2. **Break Goals into Smaller Steps**: Divide larger objectives into manageable tasks. Celebrate small victories to build momentum and confidence.

## Staying Motivated

1. **Track Your Progress**: Keep a journal of your yoga sessions, noting improvements and areas for

growth. This reflection fosters a sense of achievement.

2. **Visualize Success**: Imagine reaching your goals. Visualization reinforces commitment and encourages perseverance through challenges.

## Adjusting Goals as Needed

1. **Stay Flexible**: Life changes and unexpected events may require adjustments to your goals. Be adaptable and willing to revise objectives to maintain progress.

2. **Reflect Regularly**: Periodically review your goals to ensure they remain relevant and aligned with your evolving needs and capabilities.

## Benefits of Realistic Goals

1. **Enhanced Motivation**: Achievable goals boost confidence and motivation, reducing the risk of burnout or giving up.

2. **Improved Outcomes**: Realistic targets lead to sustainable progress and lasting benefits, enhancing your overall health and well-being.

## Common Pitfalls and How to Avoid Them

1. **Avoid Comparison**: Focus on your unique journey rather than comparing yourself to others. Everyone progresses at their own pace.

2. **Prevent Overcommitment**: Ensure goals are compatible with your lifestyle. Balance yoga with other responsibilities to maintain harmony and reduce stress.

## Encouragement and Support

1. **Build a Support Network**: Engage with friends, family, or online communities who share your interest in chair yoga. Their support can boost motivation and accountability.

2. **Seek Professional Guidance**: Consider consulting a yoga instructor for personalized advice and encouragement. They can help tailor your practice to better suit your goals.

# CHAPTER 5

# NUTRITION AND LIFESTYLE INTEGRATION

## Complementary Eating Plans for Chair Yoga

Enhancing your chair yoga practice with a complementary eating plan can accelerate weight loss and improve overall well-being. Here's how to create a balanced approach to nutrition that supports your goals.

**Understanding the Connection**

1. **Nutrition and Yoga**: A balanced diet fuels your body for yoga, providing the energy needed for effective practice and recovery.

2. **Weight Management**: Combining yoga with mindful eating helps regulate weight, enhances metabolism, and supports healthy digestion.

**Key Principles of a Complementary Eating Plan**

1. **Balanced Nutrition**: Focus on a variety of foods to ensure you're getting essential nutrients. Prioritize whole grains, lean proteins, healthy fats, and plenty of fruits and vegetables.

2. **Hydration**: Water is crucial for maintaining energy levels and aiding digestion. Aim to drink at least eight glasses a day.

## Building a Personalized Eating Plan

1. **Assess Dietary Needs**: Consider your dietary restrictions and preferences. Personalize your eating plan to fit your lifestyle and nutritional requirements.

2. **Set Realistic Goals**: Establish clear and achievable dietary objectives, such as incorporating more vegetables or reducing sugar intake.

## Incorporating Mindful Eating

1. **Listen to Your Body**: Pay attention to hunger and fullness cues. Eat when you're hungry and stop when you're satisfied.

2. **Savor Each Bite**: Slow down and appreciate the flavors and textures of your food. This practice can enhance satisfaction and prevent overeating.

**Sample Meal Ideas**

1. **Breakfast**: Start your day with oatmeal topped with fresh berries and a sprinkle of nuts for sustained energy.

2. **Lunch**: Enjoy a colorful salad with mixed greens, grilled chicken, avocado, and a light vinaigrette.

3. **Dinner**: Opt for grilled fish with a side of quinoa and steamed vegetables, offering a balanced mix of protein and fiber.

4. **Snacks**: Choose nutritious options like yogurt, nuts, or sliced fruits to keep energy levels stable throughout the day.

**Tips for Success**

1. **Plan Ahead**: Prepare meals in advance to avoid unhealthy last-minute choices. Keep your kitchen stocked with nutritious ingredients.

2. **Stay Consistent**: Make gradual changes rather than drastic dietary shifts. Consistency is key to long-term success.

## Benefits of a Complementary Eating Plan

1. **Enhanced Energy**: Proper nutrition supports your yoga practice, helping you maintain focus and stamina.

2. **Improved Digestion**: A balanced diet can alleviate digestive issues, making you feel lighter and more comfortable during practice.

3. **Weight Management**: Combining yoga with mindful eating encourages sustainable weight loss and promotes a healthy body composition.

## Avoiding Common Pitfalls

1. **Restrictive Diets**: Avoid extreme diets that can lead to nutrient deficiencies. Instead, focus on moderation and variety.

2. **Emotional Eating**: Be aware of emotional triggers that lead to overeating. Use yoga and mindfulness techniques to manage stress and emotions.

## Integrating Yoga and Nutrition

1. **Create Rituals**: Develop a pre-yoga meal routine that energizes without weighing you down. Consider light, nutritious snacks before practice.

2. **Reflect and Adjust**: Regularly assess how your eating plan impacts your yoga practice and overall well-being. Make adjustments as needed.

## Encouragement and Support

1. **Seek Guidance**: Consult a nutritionist or dietitian for personalized advice and support. They can help tailor a plan to meet your specific needs.

2. **Engage with Community**: Share your journey with others pursuing similar goals. A supportive community can provide motivation and accountability.

# Mindful Eating Techniques

Embracing mindful eating techniques can transform your relationship with food, enhancing both your physical health and mental well-being. By focusing on the present moment and tuning into your body's signals, you can develop healthier eating habits and enjoy your meals more fully.

## Understanding Mindful Eating

Mindful eating is about awareness. It's the practice of paying full attention to your eating experiences, both inside and outside the body. This involves noticing the colors, smells, textures, flavors, temperatures, and even the sounds of your food. It also includes recognizing your body's hunger and fullness signals.

## The Benefits of Mindful Eating

1. **Improved Digestion**: When you eat mindfully, you chew more slowly, which aids in digestion and allows your body to better absorb nutrients.

2. **Weight Management**: By listening to your body's hunger cues, you're less likely to overeat, helping maintain a healthy weight.

3. **Enhanced Enjoyment**: Mindful eating encourages you to savor your food, making meals more satisfying and reducing the need for larger portions.

**Practical Techniques for Mindful Eating**

**1. Set the Scene**

- **Create a Calm Environment**: Eat without distractions. Turn off the TV, put away your phone, and focus solely on your meal.

- **Appreciate the Meal**: Before you start eating, take a moment to appreciate the food in front of you. Consider its journey from farm to table.

**2. Engage Your Senses**

- **Notice the Details**: Look at the colors, textures, and arrangement of your food. Notice the aromas and imagine the flavors before taking your first bite.

- **Chew Thoroughly**: Chew each bite slowly and thoroughly. Pay attention to the textures and flavors that unfold in your mouth.

## 3. Listen to Your Body

- **Recognize Hunger and Fullness**: Check in with your body to determine your hunger level before eating. Stop when you feel comfortably full, not stuffed.

- **Differentiate Cravings from Hunger**: Ask yourself if you're eating out of true hunger or emotional cravings.

## 4. Eat Slowly

- **Pace Yourself**: Put your utensils down between bites. This slows the pace of eating and gives your body time to signal when it's full.

- **Take Small Bites**: Focus on enjoying smaller portions and extending the dining experience.

## 5. Reflect on Your Meal

- **Consider Your Mood**: Notice any emotions that arise while eating. Are you eating because you're hungry, or are you stressed or bored?

- **Practice Gratitude**: End your meal with a moment of gratitude for the nourishment it provides and the hands that helped prepare it.

## Holistic Health Tips

Embracing holistic health means considering the whole person—mind, body, and spirit—on your journey to wellness. By integrating these aspects, you can achieve balance and enhance your overall quality of life. Here are some essential tips to guide you:

**Mindful Practices**

**1. Meditation and Mindfulness**

- **Daily Meditation**: Set aside a few minutes each day to meditate. Focus on your breath and clear your mind. This practice reduces stress and enhances mental clarity.

- **Mindfulness in Action**: Be present in everyday activities. Whether eating, walking, or working, focus on the task at hand to cultivate a sense of peace and awareness.

**Physical Well-Being**

## 2. Regular Exercise

- **Find What You Love**: Choose activities that you enjoy, whether it's yoga, dancing, or walking. Consistency is key, so make exercise a fun part of your routine.

- **Balance and Flexibility**: Incorporate exercises like tai chi or Pilates to improve flexibility and balance, reducing the risk of injury and enhancing physical health.

## 3. Nutrient-Rich Diet

- **Whole Foods Focus**: Prioritize whole, unprocessed foods. Include a variety of fruits, vegetables, whole grains, and lean proteins to nourish your body.

- **Hydration**: Drink plenty of water throughout the day to stay hydrated and support bodily functions.

**Emotional and Spiritual Health**

**4. Connect with Nature**

- **Outdoor Activities**: Spend time in nature to boost your mood and reduce stress. Activities like hiking, gardening, or simply sitting in a park can have profound effects on your well-being.

- **Nature as Therapy**: Use the calming presence of nature as a form of therapy to clear your mind and rejuvenate your spirit.

**5. Cultivate Positive Relationships**

- **Social Connections**: Surround yourself with supportive, positive people. Healthy relationships can improve mental health and provide emotional support.

- **Communication**: Practice open and honest communication with loved ones to strengthen bonds and resolve conflicts.

**Mental Wellness**

**6. Continuous Learning**

- **Stimulate Your Mind**: Engage in activities that challenge your brain, like reading, puzzles, or learning a new skill. Lifelong learning keeps your mind sharp and engaged.

- **Embrace Creativity**: Explore creative outlets such as painting, writing, or music to express emotions and enhance mental well-being.

**Integrative Health Practices**

**7. Holistic Therapies**

- **Alternative Treatments**: Consider integrative therapies like acupuncture, massage, or aromatherapy. These can complement traditional treatments and promote healing.

- **Personalized Care**: Work with holistic health practitioners to create a personalized wellness plan that suits your unique needs and goals.

# CHAPTER 6

# OVERCOMING CHALLENGES

## Addressing Common Obstacles

Starting on a journey towards health and wellness often comes with its share of challenges. Recognizing and addressing these common obstacles can pave the way for a smoother path to success. Here are some strategies to overcome these hurdles effectively:

**Motivation and Consistency**

**1. Finding Motivation**

- **Set Clear Goals**: Define what you want to achieve. Whether it's losing weight, gaining strength, or improving flexibility, having a clear target helps maintain focus.

- **Visual Reminders**: Keep reminders of your goals in visible places, like sticky notes on the fridge or a vision board, to inspire daily commitment.

## 2. Building Consistency

- **Create a Routine**: Establish a daily or weekly schedule for your wellness activities. Consistency turns actions into habits, making them easier to stick with over time.

- **Track Progress**: Use a journal or app to track your achievements. Seeing progress, no matter how small, boosts motivation and reinforces positive behavior.

## Time Management

## 3. Prioritizing Health

- **Schedule Wellness**: Treat your health routines like important appointments. Allocate specific times for exercise, meal prep, and relaxation to ensure they become non-negotiable parts of your day.

- **Efficient Workouts**: Opt for short, effective workouts if time is limited. High-intensity interval training (HIIT) or quick yoga sessions can fit into even the busiest schedules.

**Physical Barriers**

## 4. Dealing with Physical Limitations

- **Modify Exercises**: Adapt exercises to suit your abilities. Use modifications to accommodate injuries or limitations, ensuring a safe and effective practice.

- **Professional Guidance**: Consult with healthcare professionals or fitness experts to tailor routines that align with your physical capabilities.

**Mental Roadblocks**

## 5. Overcoming Self-Doubt

- **Positive Affirmations**: Practice positive self-talk to counteract negative thoughts. Remind yourself of your strengths and past achievements to boost confidence.

- **Mindfulness Practices**: Engage in mindfulness or meditation to cultivate awareness and reduce anxiety. A calm mind can better tackle obstacles as they arise.

**Lifestyle Challenges**

**6. Balancing Social Influences**

- **Healthy Social Circles**: Surround yourself with supportive individuals who share your wellness goals. Positive reinforcement from peers can encourage perseverance.

- **Manage Temptations**: Plan for social events by choosing healthier options and allowing occasional indulgences without guilt.

**Emotional Well-being**

**7. Handling Stress and Setbacks**

- **Stress Management**: Incorporate stress-reducing activities like yoga, deep breathing, or journaling. These practices help maintain emotional equilibrium.

- **Learn from Setbacks**: View setbacks as learning opportunities rather than failures. Reflect on what went wrong, adjust your approach, and move forward with renewed determination.

## Staying Motivated and Consistent

Staying motivated and consistent is a transformative journey that demands more than fleeting enthusiasm; it requires a deep-seated commitment to your goals. Imagine motivation as a fire that needs constant tending. To keep the flames burning brightly, establish a robust foundation of purpose. Begin by setting clear, achievable milestones that align with your broader aspirations. These mini-victories act as stepping stones, propelling you forward and fueling your drive.

Next, cultivate a daily routine that intertwines your goals with your everyday life. Rituals, whether they're a morning meditation, a strategic to-do list, or a brief workout, serve as anchors that stabilize your focus. Track your progress meticulously; seeing how far you've come is a powerful motivator in itself. Additionally, embrace the power of accountability by sharing your journey with a supportive community or a mentor. Their encouragement and feedback can provide invaluable perspectives and keep you on track.

Finally, reward yourself for milestones achieved. Celebrating small victories creates positive reinforcement, making the pursuit of your goals more enjoyable. Remember, consistency isn't about perfection; it's about persistently making progress. Embrace the process with patience and resilience, and watch as your efforts blossom into remarkable achievements.

## Building a Supportive Community

Building a supportive community is akin to crafting a vibrant tapestry, where each thread of connection weaves a rich and intricate pattern of shared goals and mutual encouragement. Begin by identifying spaces where like-minded individuals gather—whether it's online forums, local groups, or specialized workshops. Seek out those who resonate with your values and aspirations, creating a foundation of trust and camaraderie.

Foster these connections by being genuinely present and actively participating in discussions. Share your experiences, offer your insights, and be open to receiving support and feedback. Authenticity is key; let your true self shine through, as this attracts individuals who genuinely connect with your journey.

To nurture these relationships, establish regular touchpoints. Organize meet-ups, virtual hangouts, or collaborative projects that allow members to engage meaningfully. Recognize and celebrate each other's achievements, no matter how small. This practice not only strengthens bonds but also reinforces a collective sense of purpose.

Ultimately, a supportive community thrives on reciprocity. Be prepared to both give and receive, offering a helping hand when needed and leaning on others during challenging times. By building this network of encouragement and understanding, you create a powerful, resilient circle that elevates everyone's potential and drives collective success.

# CHAPTER 7

# LONG-TERM SUCCESS

## Maintaining Progress

Maintaining progress is much like steering a ship through ever-changing seas—it requires vigilance, adaptability, and a steady hand. The key to sustaining momentum lies not just in celebrating achievements but in systematically reinforcing the habits and strategies that drive continued success.

First, cultivate a mindset of proactive reflection. Regularly assess your journey by setting aside time to review your goals and the steps you've taken towards them. This reflection should be both analytical and motivational. Analyze what strategies have worked, what obstacles you've encountered, and how your objectives may have evolved. Use this insight to adjust your approach, ensuring that your actions remain aligned with your long-term vision.

Next, create a dynamic plan that incorporates flexibility. While it's essential to have a structured roadmap, be prepared to adapt your course as circumstances change. This adaptability prevents stagnation and keeps you agile in the face of new opportunities or challenges. Incorporate short-term goals and checkpoints within your plan to provide frequent feedback loops and maintain a clear sense of direction.

Consistency is another cornerstone of progress. Establishing daily or weekly rituals—whether they are focused work periods, reflection sessions, or progress tracking—helps to anchor your efforts. These routines should be designed to fit seamlessly into your life, making it easier to adhere to them consistently. Remember, consistency does not equate to rigidity; it means maintaining a reliable rhythm that keeps you steadily advancing.

Moreover, leverage accountability mechanisms to reinforce your commitment. Sharing your goals and progress with a trusted friend, mentor, or community can provide additional motivation and insight. Regular check-ins with these individuals create a system of external encouragement and support, offering both a sounding board and a source of inspiration.

Celebrate milestones with intention. Recognize and reward yourself for reaching key achievements, no matter how small. This practice not only boosts morale but also reinforces positive behavior, making it easier to maintain focus and enthusiasm. Rewards should be meaningful to you, serving as a powerful incentive to continue progressing.

Lastly, embrace the power of resilience. Progress is rarely linear; setbacks are an inherent part of any journey. Approach challenges with a problem-solving mindset and view them as opportunities for growth. By maintaining a resilient attitude and adjusting your strategies as needed, you ensure that temporary obstacles do not derail your overall progress.

## Embracing Lifelong Wellness

Embracing lifelong wellness is an empowering journey that transcends fleeting trends and superficial goals. It's about cultivating a harmonious balance of physical vitality, mental clarity, and emotional resilience that sustains you throughout your entire life.

Begin by nurturing a holistic approach to health that integrates mindful eating, regular physical activity, and restorative rest. Choose foods that nourish both body and soul, engage in exercises that invigorate you, and prioritize sleep as a cornerstone of well-being. These fundamental practices lay the groundwork for enduring wellness.

Mental and emotional health are equally crucial. Develop habits that foster a positive mindset, such as daily gratitude practices or mindfulness meditation. Surround yourself with supportive relationships that enrich your life and provide a safe space for growth and healing.

Regular self-reflection helps you stay attuned to your evolving needs and aspirations. Set aside time to evaluate your wellness journey, adjusting your practices to align with your current life stage and goals.

Embrace wellness not as a destination, but as a lifelong adventure. By weaving together these elements into the fabric of your daily life, you create a resilient foundation for a vibrant, fulfilling existence.

## Inspirational Success Stories

Inspirational success stories are powerful narratives that illuminate the extraordinary potential within us all. These stories are not mere tales of triumph but beacons of hope, resilience, and relentless pursuit of dreams. They remind us that greatness often arises from the most unlikely beginnings, fueled by passion, perseverance, and an unwavering belief in one's potential.

Consider the journey of individuals who, against all odds, transformed their lives through sheer determination. Take, for instance, the story of a small-town entrepreneur who started with a single idea and a modest investment but through tireless effort and innovative thinking, scaled a global enterprise. Their journey is a testament to the power of vision and hard work.

Or reflect on the path of a young athlete who faced numerous setbacks and injuries but used each challenge as a stepping stone to refine their skills and achieve greatness on the world stage. Their story exemplifies the resilience needed to overcome obstacles and reach new heights.

These stories captivate us because they resonate deeply with our own aspirations and struggles. They serve as reminders that success is not a distant dream but a journey paved with courage, adaptability, and perseverance. Embracing these narratives inspires us to forge ahead, knowing that our own story is still being written, filled with endless possibilities.

# CONCLUSION

**Remember Sarah? The woman who felt trapped by her weight and limited mobility?** The one who feared exercise was out of reach? Sarah is now a shining example of what's possible. With chair yoga, she reclaimed her strength, flexibility, and confidence. Her journey wasn't about deprivation or struggle – it was about joyful movement and self-discovery.

If you've ever felt stuck, like your body is holding you back, know this: chair yoga is your key to unlocking a new chapter. It's not just about shedding pounds (though that's often a welcome side effect). It's about reigniting your energy, finding inner peace, and rediscovering what your body is truly capable of.

**Why Trust This Path?**

As a certified yoga instructor and someone who's personally witnessed the transformative power of chair yoga, I've poured my expertise and passion into this book. Every pose, every modification, and every tip is designed with your success in mind.

## The Rewards Await

By embracing chair yoga, you're not just choosing a workout routine. You're choosing:

- **Increased Strength and Flexibility:** Gentle movements build muscle and improve range of motion, even if you're starting from scratch.

- **Reduced Pain and Stiffness:** Chair yoga is incredibly therapeutic for joints and chronic conditions.

- **Boosted Energy and Mood:** The mind-body connection of yoga leaves you feeling revitalized and happier.

- **Weight Loss Support:** Increased activity, combined with the mindful eating practices encouraged in this book, creates a powerful formula for healthy weight management.

## Your Success Stories

Sarah is just one of many. Countless individuals have used this book to transform their lives. They've shared stories of pain relief, newfound confidence, and a renewed zest for life.

## Your Turn to Shine

The time for waiting is over. Your body is ready to move, to stretch, to thrive. With every page of this book, you're one step closer to the vibrant, healthy life you deserve. Don't let another day go by feeling limited.

## Thank You

Thank you for joining me on this chair yoga journey. I'm honored to have been your guide. If you've found this book valuable and inspiring, I'd be deeply grateful if you'd consider leaving a 5-star review. Your feedback helps others discover the joy of chair yoga too.